CLEAR SKIN CUISINE:

Nourishing Your Way to Pimple-Free Perfection

By

Dr. Kennedy Anakpu

TABLE OF CONTENT

INTRODUCTION

Historically, dietary modifications have received minimal attention in dermatological therapy. However, recent studies have unearthed a robust correlation between various dermatological conditions and dietary choices. Nutritional therapy is now being considered as a viable option for addressing acne, with alterations in diet potentially serving as a preventive measure against skin diseases such as aging, acne, psoriasis, and skin cancer.

The constituents of food, referred to as nutrients, play a vital role in building and sustaining body organs, supporting numerous metabolic processes, and generating energy. Adequate nutrition is crucial for the proper functioning of the skin's epidermis and dermis. Any dietary imbalance, whether it be nutritional deficiency, insufficient nutrients, excess intake, or exposure to toxic components, can disrupt the skin's equilibrium.

Deficiencies in vitamins, minerals, and fatty acids can manifest as observable cutaneous symptoms, leading to potential metabolic disturbances and dietary deficits.

WHAT IS ACNE?

Acne is a dermatological issue characterized by the formation of various types of bumps on the skin's surface, commonly appearing on the face, neck, back, and shoulders.

Hormonal changes, particularly during puberty, often serve as triggers for acne. While acne may naturally subside, it can also persist, and serious cases are associated with a heightened risk of anxiety, depression, suicidal thoughts, social phobias, and low self-esteem.

Treatment options for acne vary based on severity, ranging from no intervention to over-the-counter or prescription medications.

CAUSES OF ACNE

Understanding the development of acne involves insights into skin anatomy. The skin's surface is perforated with small holes connecting to sebaceous glands beneath the skin, known as pores. These glands produce sebum, an oily liquid, which travels to the skin's surface through thin channels called follicles. Sebum assists in eliminating dead skin cells, with a thin piece of hair growing up through the follicle.

Acne occurs when skin pores become clogged with dead skin cells, excess oil, and occasionally bacteria. Hormonal fluctuations during puberty often lead to increased oil production, elevating the risk of acne.

Two primary types of acne include:

✓   Whiteheads (closed pores protruding from the skin) and,

✓   Blackheads (open pores with tiny dark spots).

Additional types include pustules and papules.

Dietary choices can impact skin health, as certain foods prompt rapid increases in blood sugar levels. Elevated blood sugar releases insulin-like growth factor 1 (IGF-1), a hormone influencing growth effects. Excess IGF-1 in the bloodstream can stimulate oil glands to produce more sebum, thereby increasing the risk of acne and inflammation.

Certain foods, categorized as high-glycemic carbohydrates, are composed of simple sugars, including;

✓   Pasta

✓   white rice

✓   white bread

✓   and sugar

While there is a belief that chocolate may exacerbate acne, there is insufficient high-quality research to confirm this.

Foods believed to promote skin health are those with low-glycemic, complex carbohydrates such as:

✓   whole grains

✓   Legumes

✓   Unprocessed fruits and vegetables.

Additionally, skin-friendly ingredients include:

✓   Mineral zinc

✓   Vitamins A and E

✓   Antioxidants.

Examples of beneficial foods for the skin encompass:

✓   Yellow and orange fruits and vegetables (e.g., carrots, apricots, and sweet potatoes)

✓   Dark green leafy vegetables

- ✓ Tomatoes

- ✓ Blueberries

- ✓ Whole-wheat bread

- ✓ Brown rice

- ✓ Quinoa

- ✓ Turkey

- ✓ Pumpkin seeds

- ✓ Beans

- ✓ Peas

- ✓ Lentil

- ✓ Fatty fish (like salmon and mackerel)

- ✓ Nuts.

Individual responses to dietary changes vary, and some people may experience more acne when consuming certain foods. Under the supervision of a healthcare professional, experimenting with one's diet is recommended to determine what works best. It is crucial to consider any food allergies or sensitivities when planning dietary adjustments.

Vitamin A plays a vital role in skin health, and its deficiency can result in abnormal visual adaptation to darkness, as well as dry skin, hair, and brittle fingernails. This nutrient, stored in the liver, is present in the skin, particularly in the sebaceous glands expressing retinoid receptors. Dermatologists often recommend taking isotretinoin with fatty foods, as retinol (Vitamin A), carotenoids (provitamin A), and retinoids (Vitamin A metabolites) are better absorbed with simultaneous intake of vegetable oils.

The possibility that diet affects acne cannot be ruled out, especially when considering its influence on nutrient absorption and the efficacy of drugs in disease mitigation. While nutrition may not directly treat acne, it can influence its severity. While no single food is identified as a direct cause or treatment for acne, it can be asserted that certain foods may ameliorate or worsen its severity.

CHAPTER ONE

UNDERSTANDING CLEAR SKIN NUTRITION

Achieving clear and healthy skin requires a proper balance of essential nutrients, as your skin functions as a protective barrier against external elements. Nourishing your skin internally is crucial for maintaining its appearance, functionality, and overall well-being.

Healthy Fats

The radiant quality of your skin, often referred to as its "glow," is closely linked to the presence of adequate healthy fats in your diet. Insufficient fat intake can lead to dry and wrinkled skin. Prioritize monounsaturated and polyunsaturated fats sourced from plants like nuts, seeds, avocados, and fish. These fats contribute to keeping your skin moisturized, firm, and flexible, while also promoting heart health compared to saturated fats. Omega-3 fatty acids, a type of polyunsaturated fat, are essential for building cell walls, inhibiting the growth and spread of skin cancer, and potentially reducing inflammation.

Protein

Proteins from your diet are converted into amino acids, serving as building blocks for various bodily proteins, including collagen and keratin that form the structural foundation of your skin. Amino acids play a crucial role in shedding old skin.

Additionally, certain amino acids act as antioxidants, safeguarding skin cells from UV rays and free radicals generated during the breakdown of specific foods or exposure to cigarette smoke.

Vitamin A

Vitamin A is indispensable for both the upper and lower layers of the skin. It functions to prevent sun damage by interrupting collagen breakdown, offering some protection against sunburn (though not a substitute for sunscreen). Vitamin A supports the function of oil glands around hair follicles and aids in the healing process of cuts and scrapes, particularly when undergoing steroid treatment to reduce inflammation. Inadequate vitamin A levels may result in dryness, itchiness, or rough skin.

Vitamin C

Associating "C" with collagen, vitamin C plays a vital role in maintaining the structure of the protein. It acts as a potent antioxidant, shielding the skin from free radicals and potentially reducing the risk of skin cancer. Low levels of vitamin C may lead to symptoms such as easy bruising, bleeding gums, and delayed wound healing.

Vitamin E

Functioning as an antioxidant and anti-inflammatory agent, Vitamin E has the ability to absorb UV light energy, thereby preventing skin damage that may lead to wrinkles, sagging, and skin cancer. It collaborates with Vitamin C to fortify cell walls.

Zinc

Zinc, an essential mineral for optimal skin health, plays a crucial role in transporting Vitamin A, wound healing, regulating sebum production, and facilitating enzymatic activity, influencing the skin's ability to shed old cells. Due to widespread zinc deficiency in modern soil, it is recommended, especially for individuals dealing with acne, eczema, or other inflammatory skin conditions, to consider taking a zinc supplement.

Foods to Avoid

Milk and Dairy Products Milk and dairy products are often considered detrimental to skin health due to their high hormone levels, promoting oil production and leading to clogged pores. This includes familiar items such as;

✓ milk,

✓ butter,

✓ ice cream,

✓ cheese,

✓ yogurt,

✓ cream,

✓ curd.

Non-dairy alternatives are recommended to enjoy similar experiences without potential skin consequences.

Alcoholic Beverages

Alcohol, being inflammatory, exacerbates existing skin conditions, including acne, by causing more breakouts. Additionally, alcoholic beverages often contain sugary additives, compounding the pro-inflammatory effects.

Alcohol's dehydrating impact prompts increased oil production, contributing to breakouts.

Refined Carbohydrates

Including items like bread, sugar, white rice, and white flour, refined carbohydrates promote inflammation, which is unfavorable for individuals with acne-prone skin. This can lead to increased frequency and duration of acne outbreaks.

High-Glycemic Foods

Certain high-glycemic foods, such as;

✓ potatoes,

✓ parsnips,

✓ carrots,

✓ watermelon, contribute to inflammation and make it challenging to control acne. Despite appearing healthy, these foods can cause significant fluctuations in blood glucose levels, exacerbating inflammation.

Instead, opt for fruits and vegetables with lower glycemic index numbers to better manage blood glucose levels, promoting skin health.

To promote skin health and avoid wild fluctuations in blood glucose levels, consider incorporating the following foods into your diet:

- ✓ Broccoli

- ✓ Brussels sprouts

- ✓ Cauliflower

- ✓ Artichokes

- ✓ Asparagus

- ✓ Leafy greens

- ✓ Beans

- ✓ Watercress

- ✓ Radishes

- ✓ Water chestnuts

These foods are known to be skin-friendly and do not contribute to significant blood glucose fluctuations.

Foods to Avoid:

Fatty Foods

Fried and processed foods containing trans fats may contain cytokines, leading to skin redness and blotchiness, creating an environment conducive to blemishes.

Whey Protein Powder

Whey protein powder can elevate amino acids, contributing to acne formation. Studies have suggested a correlation between whey protein consumption and acne outbreaks, especially among male athletes.

Highly Processed Convenience Foods

Foods with ingredients promoting skin inflammation, unhealthy fats, and refined sugars can exacerbate acne, despite their convenience and budget-friendly nature.

Chocolate

While the main ingredient in chocolate is not the primary culprit, milk chocolate and lighter chocolates are associated with promoting acne. Dark chocolate, with less refined sugar and milk, is considered a better choice.

Chicken

Like dairy chicken may contain added hormones that could trigger inflammation, making the skin more susceptible to breakouts.

Coffee

For some, the added sugar and dairy in coffee may pose a problem, while for others, the adrenaline rush from morning coffee can boost cortisol levels, contributing to increased oil production and acne.

While making dietary changes can potentially improve acne by supporting the immune system and overall health, there is currently insufficient substantial evidence to confirm that specific foods directly cause acne. For individuals struggling with persistent acne, in addition to dietary adjustments, consulting a doctor for suitable acne treatments is advisable.

CHAPTER TWO

CONSTRUCTING A PIMPLE-FIGHTING PLATE

Fatty Fish

Fatty fish like salmon, mackerel, and herring are stellar choices for promoting healthy skin due to their richness in omega-3 fatty acids.

These essential fatty acids play a crucial role in maintaining skin thickness, suppleness, and moisture.

An omega-3 deficiency can result in dry skin. Moreover, the omega-3 fats in fish possess anti-inflammatory properties, reducing redness and acne while rendering the skin less sensitive to harmful UV rays. Studies suggest that fish oil supplements may combat inflammatory and autoimmune skin conditions like psoriasis and lupus.

Fatty fish also serves as a source of vitamin E, a vital antioxidant protecting the skin against damage from free radicals and inflammation.

Additionally, it provides high-quality protein essential for maintaining skin strength and integrity. Fish is a valuable source of zinc, regulating inflammation, overall skin health, and the production of new skin cells. A deficiency in zinc can lead to skin inflammation, lesions, and delayed wound healing.

Avocados

Avocados, rich in healthy fats, offer numerous benefits to skin health. Adequate consumption of these fats is vital for keeping the skin flexible and moisturized.

A study involving over 700 women revealed that a high intake of total fat, particularly the healthy fats found in avocados, was associated with more supple and resilient skin.

Avocados also contain compounds that may protect the skin from sun damage, preventing wrinkles and signs of aging. Moreover, avocados are a good source of vitamin E, a crucial antioxidant safeguarding the skin from oxidative damage.

Vitamin E is more effective when combined with vitamin C, another essential nutrient for healthy skin.

Vitamin C plays a key role in collagen synthesis, the primary structural protein supporting skin strength and health. A deficiency in vitamin C can result in dry, rough, and scaly skin prone to bruising. Vitamin C also acts as an antioxidant, protecting the skin from oxidative damage caused by the sun and environmental factors, which can lead to aging signs. A 100-gram serving of avocado provides 14% of the Daily Value (DV) for vitamin E and 11% of the DV for vitamin C.

Walnuts

Walnuts possess qualities that make them an exceptional food for promoting healthy skin. They are a rich source of essential fatty acids, including omega-3 and omega-6 fatty acids, which are crucial for skin health. While an excess of omega-6 fats may contribute to inflammation, omega-3 fats have anti-inflammatory properties, helping to alleviate skin conditions like psoriasis. Walnuts, with their balanced ratio of these fatty acids, may counteract the inflammatory response caused by excessive omega-6 intake.

Additionally, walnuts provide essential nutrients for proper skin function and health. A one-ounce (28 grams) serving contains 8% of the Daily Value (DV) for zinc, an essential mineral vital for skin barrier function, wound healing, and defense against bacteria and inflammation. Walnuts also supply small amounts of antioxidants such as vitamin E and selenium, along with 4–5 grams of protein per ounce (28 grams).

INCORPORATING ANTIOXIDANT-RICH FOOD

Antioxidants play a crucial role in combatting skin aging, protecting the skin from environmental factors like sun exposure and pollution. Free radicals, harmful molecules generated by environmental stressors, can damage cells, contributing to the development of fine lines, wrinkles, and age spots.

Antioxidants neutralize free radicals, preventing cellular damage and improving skin texture. They also help reduce oxidative stress, a major cause of acne and breakouts, promoting a youthful appearance. Some antioxidant-rich foods include:

Broccoli

Broccoli, a cruciferous vegetable, contains vitamins A and C. Vitamin A promotes skin health and scar reduction, while vitamin C aids in collagen production.

Broccoli also provides B vitamins, reducing dry and flaky patches. Natural estrogens in broccoli contribute to a natural glow.

Spinach Abundant in vitamins A, C, and K, spinach aids in scar healing and dark spot reduction. Its antioxidant-rich properties cleanse the body internally, combat inflammation, and enhance overall skin health. Spinach also acts as a natural sunscreen, delaying the signs of aging.

Avocado High in antioxidants and vitamins, avocado nourishes the skin, providing a natural glow. The avocado pulp contains antioxidants such as B-carotene, lecithin, and linoleic acid, moisturizing the skin. Vitamin E in avocados aids in treating chapped lips. The fruit is also rich in vitamin C and vitamin E, essential for maintaining healthy skin and protecting against free radical damage. Avocados contain antioxidants like lutein and zeaxanthin, combating free radicals and preserving skin firmness and youthfulness.

Sweet Potatoes Rich in beta-carotene, which converts to active vitamin A (retinol), sweet potatoes support cell production and growth. Increased vitamin A intake may promote the production of healthy skin cells. Anthocyanins in sweet potatoes, flavonoid antioxidants, possess anti-aging properties and contribute to skin health.

Blueberries

Blueberries are a potent source of antioxidants that combat free radicals, safeguarding skin cells from potential harm. These berries contain anthocyanins, plant substances known for their robust antioxidant properties, and are responsible for the organic purple-blue hue of blueberries. Including blueberries in your diet is an effective way to enhance daily antioxidant intake and prevent premature aging. Blueberries can be enjoyed in various ways, such as consuming them plain, adding them to smoothies and fruit salads, combining them with Greek yogurt, or using them to make jam or sauce.

Green Tea Green tea plays a protective role against environmental stress and premature aging of the skin. It contains catechins, beneficial compounds that nourish the skin, reduce inflammation, enhance moisture retention, and improve overall suppleness.

CHAPTER THREE

HYDRATION AND ENHANCED SKIN RADIANCE

The importance of hydration in achieving flawless and radiant skin often goes unnoticed in the pursuit of skincare goals. Maintaining sufficient water intake throughout the day plays a crucial role in attaining a healthy and glowing complexion. Many skincare enthusiasts emphasize the concept of "beauty from within," attributing their clear skin to proper hydration.

It's worth noting that our skin, being the largest organ in the body, acts as a protective barrier against external aggressors, safeguarding our internal organs. Dehydration can adversely affect our skin, resulting in dryness, flakiness, and the accentuation of fine lines and wrinkles. On the contrary, well-hydrated skin manifests as plump, supple, and radiant.

Adequate water consumption contributes to flushing toxins from the body, promoting clearer and healthier skin. Hydration also plays a role in maintaining the skin's natural elasticity, reducing the risk of sagging and promoting a youthful appearance. Moreover, well-hydrated skin is less susceptible to inflammation and irritation.

Recognizing the significance of hydration for our skin, let's explore effective ways to ensure its continual moisturization and radiance.

✧ Drink Abundant Water: Strive for a minimum of 8 glasses (64 ounces) of water daily. Consistent hydration throughout the day is vital for optimal skin health. Carrying a refillable water bottle ensures convenience on the go.

✧ Utilize a Hydrating Moisturizer: Invest in a high-quality moisturizer designed to provide hydration to your skin. Look for ingredients such as hyaluronic acid or glycerin, known for attracting and retaining moisture. Apply the moisturizer after gently cleansing your face and neck.

✧ Incorporate Hydrating Face Masks: Pamper your skin with hydrating face masks once or twice a week. These masks offer an intense dose of hydration and nourishment, often containing ingredients like aloe vera, cucumber, or honey, renowned for their hydrating properties.

✧ Humidify Your Environment: Dry indoor air can strip moisture from your skin. Consider using a humidifier to add moisture to the air in your home or office, creating a more skin-friendly environment, especially in dry climates or during the winter.

✧ Protect Your Skin from the Sun: UV rays can dehydrate the skin, resulting in sunburn, premature aging, and an increased risk of skin cancer. Always wear broad-spectrum sunscreen with at least SPF 30, reapplying every two hours when exposed to the sun. This practice helps maintain the skin's moisture balance and prevents damage from harmful rays.

Benefits of Water Detox:

✓ Clear and Radiant Skin: Water detox aids in eliminating toxins that can cause acne, blemishes, and other skin issues, leaving the skin looking fresh, clear, and youthful.

✓ Improved Digestion: Adequate water intake supports digestion, preventing common issues such as constipation and bloating.

✓ Weight Loss and Metabolism Boost: Water detox can enhance metabolism, leading to more efficient calorie burning and supporting weight loss.

✓ Elevated Energy Levels: Maintaining adequate hydration through water detox practices can effectively counteract fatigue, ensuring sustained vitality throughout the day.

✓ Improved Mental Clarity: Adequate hydration is instrumental in supporting optimal brain function, enhancing focus, concentration, and overall cognitive performance.

Incorporating Water Detox into Your Daily Routine

Understanding the advantages of water detox, let's explore simple ways to integrate this practice into your everyday life:

✓ Start Your Day with Warm Lemon Water: Begin your mornings with a glass of warm lemon water. This not only helps keep your body hydrated but also supports digestion, increases your vitamin C intake, and aids in detoxifying your system.

✓ Sustain Hydration Throughout the Day: Make a conscientious effort to consume a minimum of eight glasses of water daily. Take regular sips and set reminders if necessary to ensure consistent and proper hydration.

✓ Infuse Detoxifying Elements into Your Water: Amplify the detoxifying impact of water by infusing it with natural ingredients like cucumber, mint, ginger, or berries. These additions not only introduce flavor but also offer additional health benefits.

✓ Replace Sugary Beverages with Water: Substitute sugary sodas and drinks with water to diminish overall sugar intake and endorse detoxification. Opt for sparkling water or herbal teas if a flavorful alternative is desired.

✓ Embrace Intermittent Fasting: Contemplate integrating intermittent fasting into your routine, affording your body dedicated periods for rest and detoxification. Commence with shorter fasting durations, gradually extending them over time.

✓ Hydrating Beverages for Luminous Skin: Radiant and healthy skin mirrors overall well-being. While skincare products are pivotal, nurturing the skin internally is equally essential. Consuming beverages, ranging from revitalizing juices to calming herbal teas, provides potent nutrients that hydrate, revitalize, and fortify the skin's health.

The Impact of Hydration on Skin Health and Appearance:

✓ Moisture Retention: Hydration aids the skin in retaining moisture, preventing dryness, flakiness, or roughness. Well-hydrated skin exhibits a plump, smooth, and supple appearance.

✓ Enhanced Elasticity: Appropriate hydration fortifies the skin's elasticity, rendering it more resilient and less susceptible to wrinkles and fine lines. Dehydrated skin tends to manifest signs of aging more noticeably.

✓ Improved Skin Tone: Hydrated skin tends to display a more uniform tone and texture, minimizing redness, irritation, and blotchiness, resulting in a healthier and more radiant complexion.

✓ Accelerated Healing: Hydration expedites the skin's natural healing processes, aiding in the repair of damaged skin barriers, diminishing the visibility of scars, and fostering a faster recovery from wounds or skin-related issues.

Maintaining Optimal Skin Health through Dietary Choices Contrary to common belief, the regulation of oil production is linked to adequately hydrated skin. Dehydrated skin may compensate by producing excess oil, leading to breakouts or acne. Adequate hydration acts as a preventive measure against skin conditions such as eczema, psoriasis, and dermatitis, which often worsen with dry skin.

Additionally, well-hydrated skin enhances the absorption of skincare products, allowing moisturizers, serums, and other treatments to function more effectively. Hydrated skin also serves as a protective barrier against environmental stressors, including pollutants and UV rays, minimizing potential damage.

Beverages for Healthier Skin

- ✓ Green Tea Elixir: Abundant in antioxidants known as catechins, green tea fights free radicals, promoting youthful skin and reducing inflammation. Daily consumption can contribute to maintaining skin elasticity.

- ✓ Hydrating Cucumber Infusion: Adding cucumber slices to water provides optimal hydration and supports supple skin. Cucumbers, rich in silica, strengthen the skin.

- ✓ Glowing Golden Milk: Turmeric, with anti-inflammatory and antioxidant properties, combined with warm milk and honey, supports healthy, radiant skin.

- ✓ Berry Blast Smoothie: Berries packed with vitamins and antioxidants, when blended into a smoothie with coconut water or Greek yogurt, offer a collagen-boosting treat against aging signs.
- ✓ Aloe Vera Elixir: Aloe vera juice aids detoxification, soothes inflammation, and contributes to clear skin.
- ✓ Beetroot Beauty Juice: Loaded with vitamins and minerals, beetroot's detoxifying properties purify the blood, promoting a healthy complexion.

- ✓ Lemon Water Detox: Starting the day with warm lemon water kickstarts metabolism, detoxifies the system, and supports collagen production for skin elasticity.

- ✓ Coconut Water Refresher: Rich in potassium and electrolytes, coconut water maintains skin hydration and prevents dullness induced by dehydration.
- ✓ Chia Seed Hydration: Chia seeds, rich in omega-3 fatty acids and antioxidants, contribute to healthy skin when soaked in water or added to beverages.

✓ Herbal Infusions: Chamomile, peppermint, or rooibos herbal teas offer diverse skin benefits, such as anti-inflammatory properties and soothing skin irritation.

These beverages, when incorporated into a daily routine, significantly impact skin health and appearance. However, it's essential to remember that maintaining a balanced diet, a regular skincare routine, and protecting the skin from environmental damage are equally crucial. Embrace these hydrating and nutrient-rich drinks as a complement to your skincare regimen, and witness your skin glow with vitality and radiance from within.

SEAFOOD FOR HEALTHY SKIN

As we approach the summer season, revealing more skin prompts the importance of dietary choices for a radiant and healthy glow. In addition to skincare practices, incorporating seafood into the weekly diet can significantly enhance skin, hair, and nail health.
Seafood is rich in nutrients crucial for nourishing the skin internally:

✓ Omega-3 Fatty Acids:

Fatty fish like salmon and sablefish maintain the skin's natural oil barrier, promoting moisturization and reducing dryness and inflammation.

✓ Collagen Production: Zinc and copper in seafood such as shrimp and crab support collagen production, preventing fine lines and wrinkles.

✓ Antioxidants: Selenium and vitamin E in shellfish and specific fish like halibut protect the skin from free radicals, slowing down the aging process.

✓ Hydration: Seafood's high water content contributes to skin hydration, maintaining a plump and healthy complexion.

✓ Vitamin D: Fatty fish serves as an excellent source of vitamin D, essential for skin cell growth, repair, and metabolism.

Opting for Wild-Caught Seafood provides additional benefits:

✓ Lower Contaminant Risk: Wild-caught seafood is less likely to contain harmful contaminants found in farmed seafood.

✓ Higher Nutrient Density: Wild-caught seafood is more nutrient-dense, including higher levels of omega-3 fatty acids.

✓ Eco-Friendly: Choosing wild-caught seafood supports sustainable fishing practices, benefiting both the environment and skin health.

To seamlessly integrate Wild-Caught Seafood into your diet, consider trying skin-boosting recipes such as Grilled Wild Salmon, Halibut Ceviche, Shrimp and Avocado Salad, Salmon Poke Bowl, Seared Scallops with Basil Pesto, and Tuna Stuffed Avocados. These recipes provide a savory protein source and contribute to a radiant complexion through the combined benefits of omega-3 fatty acids, collagen-boosting nutrients, antioxidants, and hydration properties found in seafood.

CHAPTER FOUR

EXPLORING THE GUT-SKIN CONNECTION

Probiotics and Their Influence on Skin Well-being

Probiotics are defined as "live microorganisms that, when administered in adequate amounts, provide a health benefit to the host." It has been suggested that maintaining gut homeostasis can positively impact skin health. Individual characteristics of intestinal microflora are influenced by diet variations, encompassing factors such as age, feeding patterns, lifestyle, interactions within the flora, and pathological conditions. The increasing availability of probiotic formulations has paved the way for incorporating them into skincare routines, skin disease prevention and treatment, and anti-aging regimens. Probiotic interventions, whether for prevention or therapy, offer efficiency without adverse side effects, presenting a promising alternative to conventional treatment methods.

As the largest organ exposed to constant physical, chemical, bacterial, and fungal challenges, the skin benefits from the potential advantages of probiotics. Numerous clinical studies highlight the specific effects of probiotics on the cutaneous system, making probiotic bacteriotherapy a promising avenue for preventing and treating skin conditions such as eczema, atopic dermatitis, acne, allergic inflammation, skin hypersensitivity, UV-induced damage, wound protection, and even cosmetic applications. This paper provides a comprehensive review of the diverse health effects of probiotics on the skin.

NOURISHING YOUR GUT FOR A VIBRANT SKIN

In the pursuit of clear and radiant skin, beauty routines often steal the spotlight. However, the key to a healthy complexion extends beyond creams and serums – it lies within your gut. Embracing a gut-friendly approach to your diet can be the secret to achieving that coveted clear skin.

Understanding the Connection Between Gut Health and Skin Clarity

Ever noticed how your skin reacts when your stomach is upset? The gut and skin share a unique relationship, akin to long-lost cousins. A content gut often translates to joyful skin, while an imbalance in gut bacteria can lead to skin issues. Nourishing your gut becomes pivotal for maintaining a radiant complexion.

Essential Nutrients for Clear and Glowing Skin

Probiotics

Acting as superheroes for gut health, probiotics are found in yogurt, kefir, and fermented foods. They play a vital role in promoting a healthy gut microbiome, contributing to clearer and happier skin.

Omega-3 Fatty Acids

Considered VIPs in the realm of skin health, omega-3 fatty acids are abundant in fatty fish, flaxseeds, and walnuts. These nutrients work behind the scenes, combating inflammation and supporting the skin's natural radiance.

Antioxidants

Think of antioxidants as bodyguards for your skin. Berries, dark chocolate, and green tea are rich sources of antioxidants, offering protection against the chaos caused by free radicals. Embracing these antioxidant-rich foods stands as a defense against the aging process, earning gratitude from your skin.

Ways to Achieve Luminous Skin through Dietary Choices

✧ Enhance your skin's radiance by incorporating fermented foods into your meals, promoting both gut health and a clear complexion. From kimchi to kombucha, these foods not only support a healthy gut but also contribute to a complexion that exudes clarity. Stay tuned for easy recipes that will delight your taste buds.

✧ Elevate your skin's clarity with a variety of vibrant fruits and vegetables, going beyond basic salads. Craft visually appealing plates that not only bid farewell to dull skin but also welcome the vibrant glow of a mango sunrise.

✧ Who says nutritious food has to be dull? Indulge in delicious recipes rich in omega-3 fatty acids, such as salmon sushi bowls and walnut pesto pasta. These tasty recipes not only cater to your palate but also bring a lively, celebratory atmosphere to your skin.

Foods to Steer Clear of for a Flawless Complexion

Exercise caution with certain foods; not all are welcome at the clear-skin party. Some foods act as unwelcome intruders, causing issues for your gut and appearing on your face uninvited. Bid farewell to these culprits for a flawless complexion.

Gut-Friendly Practices for Improved Skin

Your journey to a healthy gut extends beyond the dining table. Hydration, stress management, and regular exercise play pivotal roles in maintaining radiant skin. Keep your gut hydrated, manage stress effectively, and make exercise a regular part of your routine. This comprehensive approach will guide your gut and skin towards enduring bliss.

Lifestyle Practices for Clear Skin

A. Techniques for Stress Management:

Stress is inevitable, but prolonged and chronic stress can negatively impact your skin. Elevated stress levels release hormones like cortisol, leading to various skin issues. Effectively managing stress is crucial for maintaining skin health. Practices like mindful meditation and prioritizing adequate sleep can induce a sense of calm and support skin rejuvenation.

Tips for Managing Stress:

✓ Regular Exercise: Engage in regular, vigorous exercise to burn off cortisol and positively impact stress levels.

✓ Mindfulness: Incorporate mindfulness into your routine through activities like yoga or deep breathing exercises.

✓ Balanced Diet: Pay attention to your food choices, opting for whole foods and fresh fruits and vegetables.

✓ Mindful Eating: Eliminate distractions during meals to reduce overeating and promote weight maintenance.

✓ Body Detoxification: Cut back on toxins like alcohol and tobacco for improved well-being and clearer thinking.

✓ Encourage Endorphin Release: Engage in activities that promote endorphin release, such as physical contact or joyful activities.

✓ Pursue Happiness: Activities that bring joy contribute to a positive mood and lower stress levels.

✓ Engage in Conversation: Talking with loved ones positively influences stress levels and provides valuable support.

✓ Embrace Nature: Spending time outdoors or bringing nature indoors can offer therapeutic benefits for stress relief.

✓ Prioritize Sleep: A healthy sleep routine plays a significant role in reducing stress and supporting skin repair.

B. Importance of Sleep in Skin Repair:

Quality sleep is essential for overall well-being and energy levels, but it also plays a crucial role in skin health. Skin cells undergo repair and regeneration during sleep, contributing to the maintenance of optimal skin condition. Collagen and hyaluronic acid production, essential for youthful and glowing skin, are promoted through quality sleep. Adequate hydration and a well-functioning circulation system are also facilitated during sleep, preventing issues like dark circles and puffy skin.

Conversely, insufficient or poor-quality sleep has adverse effects on skin health. Elevated cortisol levels and impaired cell repair lead to dull, dehydrated, and stressed skin. The decrease in collagen production results in lackluster and deflated skin, contributing to premature aging. For individuals with sensitive skin, a lack of sleep can further compromise the skin's protective barrier, making it more susceptible to irritants and infections.

Premature Aging:

The skin's natural activities during sleep play a crucial role in preventing premature aging, such as fine lines, dullness, and loss of volume. Sleep deprivation negatively impacts collagen production, diminishing the skin's elasticity and contributing to sagging. Dark circles around the eyes can also appear due to poor circulation and hydration levels. Skincare products, like System D eye serum and Feather Canyon eye cream, can address specific issues such as puffy eyes and fine lines. Hyaluronic Acid, found in products like the Hydrating Booster and Back To Life serum, provides essential hydration.

CHAPTER FIVE

Meal Planning for Pimple-Free Days

Foods That Cause Acne:

Understanding the connection between diet and acne is a personalized journey, as each person reacts differently to various foods. Observing how the skin responds to different items helps identify potential breakout triggers. Generally, foods with higher sugar content can impact insulin levels, influencing other hormones linked to skin health.

◆ Sugar:

Refined sugar, present in foods like cane sugar, can contribute to acne by raising blood sugar levels and increasing insulin levels. The rapid absorption of refined carbs into the bloodstream may lead to inflammation, potentially exacerbating acne. Monitoring how the skin reacts to different foods, especially those with high sugar content, is essential in managing acne triggers.

◆ HIGH-GLYCEMIC FOODS

In addition to sugar, refined grains and white flour can cause a rapid spike in blood sugar levels. Simple carbohydrates found in white bread and pasta are easily converted into glucose, the body's energy source. Conversely, slowly-digested carbs from vegetables and whole grains have a lower glycemic index due to their fiber content. Regular consumption of high-glycemic foods without combining them with protein and healthy fats can elevate blood sugar levels, impacting hormones. Insulin, in particular, enhances the activity of androgen hormones, accelerating cell growth and sebum production, leading to acne.

◆ DAIRY PRODUCTS

All types of milk, even organic, contain hormone triggers that may contribute to acne, including precursors to testosterone and other androgens. While cow's milk and whey protein may increase the risk of acne, there is limited research supporting a direct link between dairy-derived products like yogurt or cheese and increased breakouts. For those experiencing chronic acne while consuming dairy regularly, experimenting with a temporary elimination of dairy or switching to low-glycemic milk alternatives like unsweetened almond, hemp, or coconut milk is recommended.

FOODS TO EAT FOR CLEAR SKIN

Consistently supporting your skin involves supporting your cells through a focus on consuming real, whole foods in their natural state. These foods, which have nourished humanity for thousands of years, include avocados, berries, eggs, wild-caught salmon, and sweet potatoes Emphasizing specific macro and micronutrients in an acne diet plan can contribute to clearer skin:

Complex carbohydrates:

Opt for quinoa, 100% whole wheat bread, brown rice, legumes, fruits, and starchy veggies to maintain balanced blood sugar levels.

Probiotics:

Cultivate a healthy gut by incorporating fermented foods like kefir, yogurt, tempeh, sauerkraut, and kimchi.

Turmeric:

Harness the anti-inflammatory properties of curcumin in turmeric to reduce inflammation, target pores, and promote skin calmness.

Omega-3 fatty acids:

Integrate salmon, walnuts, and flaxseed to support healthy cell membranes, acting as barriers to pollution and bacteria.

Vitamins A, C, and E:

Ensure sufficient intake of these vitamins found in various foods like tuna, mackerel, liver, cream, feta cheese, almonds, peanuts, avocados, broccoli, citrus, papaya, and tomatoes.

Zinc:

Incorporate zinc-rich foods such as legumes, beans, seeds, high-quality animal protein, and shellfish, as low zinc levels may contribute to acne.

TIPS BEFORE STARTING AN ACNE DIET PLAN

Before embarking on an acne diet plan, consider the following:

✓ Fuel up on whole foods: Consume healthy whole foods containing slow-digesting carbs, fiber, and essential fats like coconut oil and avocado.

✓ Opt for high-quality meat and dairy: Choose zinc-rich options such as red meat, fatty fish, and shellfish.

✓ Consult with a dermatologist or esthetician: Seek professional advice to ensure alignment with your skincare goals and potential food-related triggers.

7-Day Acne Diet Plan

This well-rounded and colorful acne diet plan features nourishing foods, providing a delightful and wholesome experience throughout the week. The plan includes a variety of meals designed to support skin health and overall well-being.

✓ Monday:

Commence the day with an Anti-Inflammatory Berry + Turmeric Muffin paired with two scrambled eggs cooked in ghee, coconut oil, or extra-virgin olive oil. Follow up with a nourishing Grain Bowl and indulge in a satisfying Thai Chicken Salad.

✓ Tuesday:

Savor smoked salmon with non-dairy cream cheese (options like VioLife and Kite Hill), accompanied by pickled onion and cucumber slices on a sprouted grain English muffin (opt for gluten-free if needed). Enjoy another nutritious Grain Bowl and make use of leftover Thai Chicken Salad.

✓ Wednesday:

Start the day with another round of the Anti-Inflammatory Berry + Turmeric Muffin, coupled with two scrambled eggs cooked in ghee, coconut oil, or extra-virgin olive oil. Enhance your menu with a Chocolate Green Smoothie and relish Citrus Salmon with brown rice and sautéed zucchini.

✓ Thursday:

Delight in a Tropical Pineapple Ginger Smoothie to kick off the morning, followed by a Black Lentil Salad with Roasted Veggies and Shrimp Skewers paired with Tzatziki for a flavorful day.

✓ Friday:

Repeat the morning routine with the Anti-Inflammatory Berry + Turmeric Muffin and two scrambled eggs cooked in ghee, coconut oil, or extra-virgin olive oil. Relish Turmeric Chicken Immunity Soup and treat yourself to Chimichurri Fish Tacos.

✓ Saturday:

Indulge in a Goat Cheese Frittata for a delightful start, accompanied by Turmeric Chicken Immunity Soup and a Black Lentil Salad with Roasted Veggies.

✓ Sunday:

Conclude the week with another round of Goat Cheese Frittata and a Chocolate Green Smoothie. Cap off the day with Crispy Roasted Sweet Potatoes for a delicious and wholesome meal.

Additionally, it's crucial to schedule regular visits to a dermatologist, at least once a year, even if you don't currently have specific skin concerns. Understanding the impact of diet on your skin is essential, as a healthy diet not only contributes to clearer skin but also plays a preventive role in avoiding skin cancers, such as melanoma or carcinoma.